CW01457326

CHRONIC

AFFIRMATIONS

365 Daily Affirmations for

Chronic Illness and Pain Sufferers

Written by:

Judith S. Copper

The information provided in this book is for entertainment purposes only and is not intended to be a substitute for professional medical advice, diagnosis, or treatment. Always seek the advice of a qualified healthcare provider with any questions you may have regarding a medical condition. The author and publisher of this book make no representations or warranties of any kind, express or implied, about the completeness, accuracy, reliability, suitability or availability with respect to the information, products, services, or related graphics contained in this book for any purpose. Any reliance you place on such information is therefore strictly at your own risk.

COPYRIGHT © 2023 BY JUDITH S. COPPER
CHRONIC AFFIRMATIONS: 365 Daily Affirmations for Chronic Illness and Pain Sufferers

Notice of Copyright

This book is copyright protected by the author. No part of this book may be reproduced, stored in a retrieval system, or transmitted in any form or by any means, electronic, mechanical, photocopying, recording, or otherwise, without the prior written permission of the author. This book is for personal use only and may not be resold or given away to other people.

Published by:
Rittin Books

Printed in the United States of America

First Printing Paperback Edition, 2023
ISBN 9798818141879

SPECIAL BONUS!
WANT THIS BOOK FOR FREE?

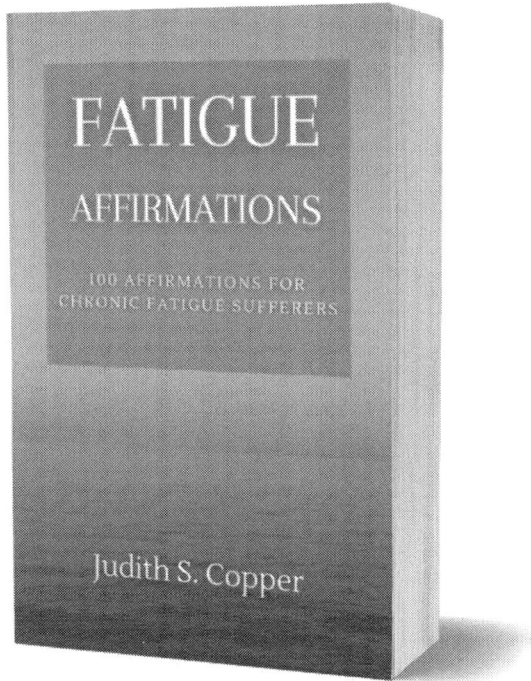

FATIGUE

AFFIRMATIONS

100 AFFIRMATIONS FOR
CHRONIC FATIGUE SUFFERERS

Judith S. Copper

Get *FREE*, unlimited access to it and all my new books by joining the Fan Base!

SCAN WITH YOUR CAMERA TO JOIN

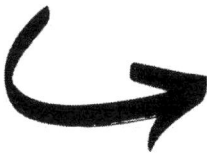

DEDICATION

This book is dedicated to anyone suffering from any form of chronic pain or chronic illness.

It's for you, me, and others like us.

I hope you find value in this book and that it will help you on your journey.

TABLE OF CONTENTS

CHRONIC AFFIRMATIONS

365 Daily Affirmations for Chronic Illness and Pain Sufferers

PREFACE

For over ten years, I have been struggling with a condition known as Ankylosing Spondylitis (AS) - a debilitating and painful chronic illness that fuses the spine and can cause a range of symptoms such as arthritis throughout the entire body, uveitis and chronic fatigue syndrome. I have faced the full range of symptoms associated with this condition, and over the years, I have struggled with intense pain, fatigue, brain fog, depression, anxiety and more. Despite the best efforts of medical professionals, the last eight years were filled with unrelenting pain and fatigue, and in 2020, I hit rock bottom.

At that time, my life was in ruins, my marriage had fallen apart, and I started developing anti-social behavior as I isolated myself from others. I turned to alcohol too often at social gatherings, and my mood was sour and negative. I am still ashamed of my behavior now, but I recognize that I was simply a victim of a terrible illness that I had left untreated for too long.

But one day, something changed within me. I felt an overwhelming urge to change and try to make the best of what I had left. I didn't know where to start, but I knew that getting out of bed was a reasonable first step. So, I did. I went to my computer and searched the internet for everything related to my condition and similar conditions with similar challenges.

I tried many different things and measured their impact on my fatigue, pain levels, and mental state. Some things helped, while others made no difference at all. Then, one day, I stumbled upon an affirmations book designed to help with depression and started reading its uplifting and empowering words.

I read the affirmations daily, repeated them many times, and soon saw their impact on my life. Focusing on the positive became more accessible, and even small tasks and daily chores seemed effortless compared to how they had felt before. Although the affirmations were intended for those dealing with mental health issues, they were also relevant to my situation. I could relate to them even though the root of my problems was not psychological.

However, I realized that many who struggle with physical health also struggle with mental health. I saw a need for a book that focused specifically on the challenges those with chronic illnesses face. So, I decided to create my own book focused on chronic disease and pain, hoping to reach others in similar situations.

Through the pages of this book, you will find the strength and courage to cope with and overcome your condition. I hope it provides comfort and inspiration, and I wish you a pleasant reading experience.

Warmest wishes,

Judith

INTRODUCTION

As individuals suffering from chronic illnesses, we often struggle with physical symptoms and the mental and emotional toll that such a condition can bring. It can be easy to become consumed by the pain, fatigue, and frustration that come with managing a chronic illness and feel as though we are simply the sum of our symptoms. However, it is essential to remember that our experiences, no matter how trying, do not define us.

We are the product of the memories, experiences, and influences that shape our thoughts and perspectives. Our experiences, both positive and negative, form the foundation of who we are and whom we will become. If we allow the hardships of chronic illness to become a defining factor in our lives, we risk becoming the illness itself.

However, this does not have to be the case. By intentionally seeking out positive experiences and reframing how we talk to and about ourselves, we can actively work to shape a more hopeful and resilient version of ourselves. It takes effort and dedication, but the rewards can be immeasurable.

Whether you are struggling with physical symptoms, mental health issues, or both, this book is a tool for finding hope and resilience in the face of adversity.

HOW TO USE THIS BOOK

To use this book effectively, it is recommended to adopt a daily routine of reading one verse daily. This allows you to focus entirely and reflect on each affirmation and how it can apply to your life.

Repeating each affirmation throughout the day is also recommended, as this helps solidify its meaning and message in your mind. This repetition can be done verbally or simply by thinking about the affirmation throughout the day.

Writing affirmations in a diary can be an excellent exercise for those who enjoy journaling. This allows you to reflect on the affirmations and how they relate to your experiences and thoughts. It can also serve as a record of your journey and growth.

Incorporating affirmations into your meditation routine can be a powerful tool for those who practice meditation. Focus on the words of the affirmation as you take deep breaths and let the message sink into your mind and heart.

By incorporating these practices into your daily routine, you can fully embrace the power and positivity of the affirmations in this book and unleash its potential to bring positive change and growth into your life.

CHRONIC AFFIRMATIONS

I think; therefore, I am

René Descartes, philosopher

I speak; therefore, I am

Andrea Moro, linguistic

I speak; therefore, I think

Francis Kemble, novelist

And through language, I perceive myself

Judith S. Copper, chronic illness sufferer

Language is a crucial component in shaping our thoughts and ideas. It is a well-established fact among social scientists and researchers that language use dramatically impacts our ability to think abstractly and understand concepts. This is why discourse theory, which examines the relationship between language and our understanding of the world, is a significant branch of social sciences.

Discourse theory is primarily concerned with the power dynamics within society and how language either supports or challenges these power structures. Prominent scholars in this field, such as Jurgen Habermas, Harold Garfinkel and Michel Foucault, have all developed their theories based on this understanding of the role of language in shaping our perceptions and thoughts.

In addition to its impact on our social understanding, language also plays a significant role in shaping our perceptions of ourselves, particularly regarding our health. Medical discourse theory, a branch of the medical sciences, explores the relationship between language, self-perception and physical health, highlighting both the positive and negative effects that language can have.

Given the similarities in the views held by both the social sciences and the medical sciences regarding the role of language in shaping our perceptions, it is reasonable to assume that language also plays a significant role in shaping our self-perceptions.

Positive affirmations are a prime example of how language can shape our perceptions. Studies have shown that positive affirmations can have a tangible impact on our thoughts and beliefs. In essence, the affirmations we read, hear or speak out loud shape our reality to a certain extent. This is why it is essential to make an effort to focus on positive self-talk, especially for individuals who struggle with chronic conditions and often question themselves.

To apply positive affirmations to your daily routine, consider incorporating them into your daily rituals. Try reading one affirmation out loud to yourself each day, and make it a habit to incorporate this into your daily routine. Doing this can positively shape your perceptions and beliefs, leading to a more fulfilling and empowering life.

JUDITH S. COPPER

January

JUDITH S. COPPER

January 1st

My affirmations make me aware of the power of my thoughts.

January 2nd

I am worthy of a joyful, happy, and purposeful life. My chronic illness does not get to steal that away from me.

January 3rd

I give love and compassion to myself.

January 4th

I am not a statistic. My story is unique.

January 5th

I will handle what life throws at me.

January 6th

I am not defined by my illness - I am a warrior.

January 7th

I make time to tend to and care for my body.

January 8th

I know how to delegate responsibilities to others in

a healthy manner.

January 9th

I prioritize and practice self-care on a daily basis.

January 10th

I will not suffer.

January 11th

My diagnosis was the starting point to build a better life.

January 12th

I ask for what I need, hold boundaries, and protect my health.

January 13th

The decisions made for me by doctors or well-meaning friends do not actually dictate my decisions.

January 14th

I am a willing participant in my own wellness plan.

January 15th

I deserve to be loved.

January 16th

I am my own best advocate.

January 17th

The couch is sometimes better than being social and that is okay.

January 18th

I will not be ashamed of my story. I will use it to inspire others.

January 19th

I am willing to be with all of my thoughts and feelings without admonishing them. Instead of turning away, I stay and understand.

January 20th

I am worthy of good health.

January 21st

I wake up each morning. It may take a bit longer than for others, but I will get up.

January 22nd

The more I listen to my body, the more my body listens to me.

January 23rd

I am not my pain.

January 24th

I release all guilt and shame about my illness.

January 25th

Pain is inevitable, suffering is a choice.

January 26th

Every choice I make, I make it with mindfulness and a love of life. Whatever it is that I do, I love myself through it.

January 27th

I am the hero of my story.

January 28th

I will do what I love to do.

January 29th

Today is not yesterday.

January 30th

I will look for ways to solve and improve my everyday responsibilities.

January 31st

I am open to seeking holistic or alternative therapies.

JUDITH S. COPPER

February

JUDITH S. COPPER

February 1st

There might not be a cure but there is a solution.

February 2nd

I will get through this.

February 3rd

I will rest when I need to.

February 4th

I have endured this discomfort before and survived it. Therefore, I will also survive it today.

February 5th

I am happy because I choose to be.

February 6th

My mind is stronger than my pain.

February 7th

I am not my illness.

February 8th

Sometimes it feels like the small things for me are
like climbing a mountain. I am proud every
mountain top I reach.

February 9th

I will not be stubborn and only rely on myself.

February 10th

When I feel like giving up, I will focus on the positive things that I have in my life.

February 11th

Pain can require a cane and that is okay. Gentlemen with high hats used to have canes and therefore I carry mine with pride like an 1800's gentleman or connoisseur.

February 12th

I will remember to have fun.

February 13th

I look back at my memories in joy of what was before I got ill. I also look at the good things that my condition has brought with it.

February 14th

I accept the help I get offered.

February 15th

I have permission to fall asleep.

February 16th

I acknowledge that my energy is limited and do not stress about things that others can sort out themselves.

February 17th

Where there is a will there's a way.

February 18th

I let all feelings flow freely through me.

February 19th

I will ask for help if needed.

February 20th

I accept that other people's problems might seem small to me though they are real problems from their perspective.

February 21st

I release all stress and negative thoughts about my condition.

February 22nd

Sometimes, when I feel like giving up, I focus on the positive things that I have in my life.

February 23rd

I chose to remain positive so that my body may heal.

February 24th

I deserve to be treated equally to my peers.

February 25th

I will let go of my chronic pain.

February 26th

I deserve kindness.

February 27th

When I do my best, it is enough.

February 28th

I will spread awareness to let others know that they are not alone.

February 29th

This day only comes around every fourth year. Like the 29th of February, people like me are special.

JUDITH S. COPPER

March

JUDITH S. COPPER

March 1st

I am an unstoppable warrior who is strong and fearless.

March 2nd

My hardships are my lessons, and I will use them to grow stronger.

March 3rd

I like myself. A lot.

March 4th

I will stop worrying about everything.

March 5th

My body may hurt but I am in control over my own
state of mind.

March 6th

I am not a disappointment. People who don't
understand are.

March 7th

I will stop at nothing.

March 8th

I know myself and I am in-tune with what I need.

March 9th

I will not give up.

March 10th

Sometimes my body breaks. When that happens, I will put the pieces back together.

March 11th

I only compare myself with myself - in that way I will grow.

March 12th

I am happy and am going to stay that way.

March 13th

I will stand up for others.

March 14th

Even when I struggle to love myself, I will pay

attention to my needs.

March 15th

I see my illness as an opportunity for a fresh start

and define myself from new.

March 16th

I am not a victim.

March 17th

I will conquer this condition and punch destiny in its face.

March 18th

Sometimes I face my fears and sometimes I don't. It is only me who decides when I feel like being brave.

March 19th

I will thrive, not just survive.

March 20th

I am courageous and fight to live each day with joy.

March 21st

Sometimes the small things feel big to me, and I offer myself compassion when they do.

March 22nd

I make regular visits within myself to remain positive.

March 23rd

It's okay to not be okay.

March 24th

Being strong is my way of life.

March 25th

I allow myself to express how I feel.

March 26th

I choose to make this day my own and to speak words that create a reality I enjoy.

March 27th

Each day has the potential for new happiness.

March 28th

I wake up each morning ready to face new challenges.

March 29th

I will find a doctor who will listen.

March 30th

I look back and see the long way of growth I have

taken.

March 31st

Today is a fresh start.

JUDITH S. COPPER

April

JUDITH S. COPPER

April 1st

I will let go of my worries, fears, and blame.

April 2nd

I am worthy of love.

April 3rd

My potential for happiness is not limited by my chronic illness

April 4th

My condition is my springboard to betterment.

April 5th

I am enough. Always.

April 6th

I do not judge people for their lack of understanding. They have not had the same experiences that I have.

April 7th

I invite all the good qualities of sleep and rest.

April 8th

I do not deserve the pain I'm in.

April 9th

Good things happen every day.

April 10th

I will work towards relieving stress and keeping a

healthy piece of mind.

April 11th

I do not let the pain change who I am.

April 12th

I will find the company in others with similar

conditions.

April 13th

I will not go down without a fight.

April 14th

I know how to look at different perspectives with

ease.

April 15th

I am grateful for my healing.

April 16th

There are good things and there are bad - I choose

to focus on the former.

April 17th

My illness does not equal my value.

April 18th

When something breaks, I choose to put it back
together like a beautiful mosaic.

April 19th

My condition does not define my personhood.

April 20th

I deserve respect.

April 21st

I am much more than my condition.

April 22nd

I will get through this.

April 23rd

Though I may be fractured, I am not fully broken

yet.

April 24th

I will be strong.

April 25th

I deserve a healthy sex life and am open to using helping aids if it comes to that.

April 26th

I'm a fighter and a survivor.

April 27th

I am ready to let go of the responsibilities that no longer serve me.

April 28th

I will not turn bitter.

April 29th

I am strong, called, capable and ready for this day.

April 30th

I recognize that others struggle with less pain than I
do and that is okay.

JUDITH S. COPPER

May

JUDITH S. COPPER

May 1st

I will be hopeful.

May 2nd

Crying is not a sign of weakness.

May 3rd

Every challenge has a hidden treasure.

May 4th

I will have a meaningful life with my chronic illness.

May 5th

Courage runs through my veins

May 6th

Though my back may be stiff my spirit stands up
straight.

May 7th

I am grateful for my healing.

May 8th

I am committed to being my best, healthiest self.

May 9th

With my hardships, I gain insight.

May 10th

I will not avoid other issues in my life.

May 11th

I am strong enough to push myself and wise enough
to know when I need resting.

May 12th

There are people out there who suffer more than
me.

May 13th

My potential for happiness is not limited by my chronic illness.

May 14th

I choose happiness over pain.

May 15th

When I fall, I always pick myself up.

May 16th

I am a warrior full of courageousness and hope.

May 17th

I can, therefore I will.

May 18th

My health challenges make me stronger.

May 19th

I know that some people are healthy. Good for them.
I will remain happy for their good health.

May 20th

I will make room for others to experience pain even
though I may be in much more pain.

May 21st

I find joy and let it burn out the pain.

May 22nd

Decisions made by doctors are ultimately my own to

make.

May 23rd

I will hold on to my good humor.

May 24th

I will be understanding and respectful when others

stress their hardships.

May 25th

Every day I learn to live and love my illness.

May 26th

My peace is more powerful than my pain.

May 27th

I see through the advice given by well-meaning friends and family members even though I might have other thoughts on their suggestions.

May 28th

With my condition, I am gaining insight.

May 29th

I appreciate each day and its opportunities.

May 30th

I am more than my condition.

May 31st

I am on the path of expansion, always learning. I respect the process even when I do not understand it.

JUDITH S. COPPER

June

JUDITH S. COPPER

June 1st

I will do this one moment at a time.

June 2nd

I know that I do the very best I can.

June 3rd

Every tickling pain and every aching joint will stop

bothering me.

June 4th

I choose to believe that one day there will be a cure.

June 5th

Through perspective I gain strength and wisdom.

June 6th

I focus deeply on my illness and lay it to rest.

June 7th

With my condition, I am growing stronger.

June 8th

I am looking for ways to express love. I am looking
for beauty in the present moment. I am looking for
beacons of hope everywhere I go.

June 9th

I am grateful for the good days.

June 10th

I will create a body that supports me.

June 11th

I do not linger in my illness.

June 12th

I do not linger in my pain.

June 13th

I am thankful for healing.

June 14th

I am strong and able to overcome all obstacles on
my path.

June 15th

I demand treatment from hospitals and will win over
its bureaucracy.

June 16th

I will accept my condition and seek the help I need.

June 17th

I will get through anything.

June 18th

I have many goals and dreams and I will achieve them.

June 19th

There are solutions. I will keep on looking and will eventually find them.

June 20th

I will not forget to treat myself as I treat others.

June 21st

Disability is nothing but a term used towards a specific thing or idea. I am not disabled. I am able, and very much at that.

June 22nd

I am in pain. Yes. But pain does not break me.

June 23rd

I will get the rest I need whenever I need it.

June 24th

I am the creator of my future.

June 25th

I am wise and have learned my wisdom the hard way. This makes me stronger and more insightful than my peers.

June 26th

I will remain hopeful and do not turn blue when hope feels lost.

June 27th

Sometimes I get hit by an avalanche of emotions. When that happens, I dig myself free again.

June 28th

I will push through.

June 29th

I might not always see the light at the end of the

tunnel, but I am able to convince myself that there

is light.

June 30th

I will prosper.

JUDITH S. COPPER

July

JUDITH S. COPPER

July 1st

I have so many good things in life to be thankful for.

July 2nd

My strongest ally is the person I see in the mirror.

July 3rd

I accept seeking advice with others.

July 4th

I am a faithful believer in myself.

July 5th

I do not sit back and let my condition take its pulls
on me.

July 6th

Though there are parts of me that are weak, I myself
am strong.

July 7th

I get up and I push through.

July 8th

I separate these obstacles from how I define myself.

July 9th

This illness is my body trying to tell me something.

July 10th

I am grateful for my amazing body.

July 11th

When I fall, I get back on my feet.

July 12th

I actively use self-care to soothe me when I'm in

pain.

July 13th

I choose happiness.

July 14th

My condition does not determine my value.

July 15th

Some people are stronger than others. I am that

person, because I have to be.

July 16th

Today is the start of something good.

July 17th

I choose to release this illness.

July 18th

I have many goals and dreams and I don't give up
until I achieve them.

July 19th

I base my happiness on my progress.

July 20th

I live each day and find joy.

July 21st

I feel peace along with my pain.

July 22nd

I will create the life I deserve.

July 23rd

Challenges are opportunities for growth.

July 24th

I get to write my own story.

July 25th

I am a friend to my body. I forgive my body and treat it with the same loving kindness I would like to receive.

July 26th

Mistakes are the starting point for success.

July 27th

I have the heart of a Warrior

July 28th

I listen to my body.

July 29th

I accept good health and healing throughout my body.

July 30th

I'm not a burden to those around me - even if they act like I am.

July 31st

I give myself permission to heal.

JUDITH S. COPPER

August

JUDITH S. COPPER

August 1st

No matter what has been or will be, my inner light
can't be extinguished.

August 2nd

My body is a temple - I will treat it with the utmost
care.

August 3rd

I choose happiness over my pain.

August 4th

I acknowledge my pain and let it go.

August 5th

I not only make lemonade, I squeeze the hell out of

life's lemons.

August 6th

I am strong, capable, and confident

August 7th

Dwelling on my limitations leads me nowhere.

August 8th

I am beautiful.

August 9th

I strive for progress, not perfection.

August 10th

I am a work in progress.

August 11th

I surround myself with people who support my

wellness journey.

August 12th

I am a dream-chaser.

August 13th

I am learning what my body needs and how to best take care of it myself.

August 14th

Tomorrow is a new day.

August 15th

I adapt to my condition and set new goals that are suitable for my situation.

August 16th

I will accomplish anything I set my mind to.

August 17th

I look back at my achievements and know that hurdles on my path are battles that will be conquered.

August 18th

I do not dwell on things that cannot be.

August 19th

I focus on myself and my own self-improvement.

August 20th

My ability to rise is stronger than my falls.

August 21st

I am strong, willful, and brave.

August 22nd

I keep myself in order and do what I must do.

August 23rd

I am open to seeking wisdom from religion or

religious teaching.

August 24th

My hard work will pay off.

August 25th

I have faith in my abilities.

August 26th

I'm not less worthy because of my disability.

August 27th

I got this.

August 28th

I release the need to punish myself and only make healthy choices from a place of love.

August 29th

I only measure myself with my former self of yesterday.

August 30th

I will make my own morning rituals.

August 31st

I consume positive information, material, entertainment, and conversations.

JUDITH S. COPPER

September

JUDITH S. COPPER

September 1st

I do not oppose my pain.

September 2nd

I laugh when I can and sing when I can.

September 3rd

I am resilient.

September 4th

I treat my discomfort and pain like I would an
innocent child. I tend to my body with
unconditional compassion and care.

September 5th

I find joy in the little things.

September 6th

I appreciate and love my body.

September 7th

The more I care for my body, the more it cares for me.

September 8th

Every day brings new opportunities for healing.

September 9th

I am open to new ways of improving my health.

September 10th

Good things happen to me because I am a good person who deserves it.

September 11th

My body is in a state of harmony.

September 12th

I choose to be healthy.

September 13th

My mind is calm and at peace.

September 14th

I am safe.

September 15th

I am loved.

September 16th

I keep my body and mind in balance by attending to
my physical and mental state.

September 17th

I grow stronger every day.

September 18th

My body supports me.

September 19th

I give thanks for what this illness has taught me.

September 20th

I treat my body with respect and compassion.

September 21ˢᵗ

With every breath I exhale I release my illness.

September 22ⁿᵈ

I am free to be new in this moment.

September 23ʳᵈ

I let go of all negative thoughts and feelings.

September 24ᵗʰ

I will seek knowledge about my prognosis and use

that knowledge for betterment.

September 25th

I will overcome it.

September 26th

I am respecting my body and doing what I can, with where I am now.

September 27th

I commit myself to feeling better.

September 28th

I will live a rich, successful life surrounded by friends and family.

September 29th

Every part of my body is ready to let go of the illness

and pain.

September 30th

I know my thoughts influence my reality.

.

October

JUDITH S. COPPER

October 1st

I will not let this illness get the best of me.

October 2nd

I am grateful to be alive.

October 3rd

I matter.

October 4th

My life has a purpose.

October 5th

I am sick and tired of being sick and tired - therefore I will act on my condition and improve my situation.

October 6th

I am listening and learning from my illness.

October 7th

I did not bring this on myself.

October 8th

I hold the vision of myself smiling, light, active and thriving.

October 9th

My pain does not result in suffering.

October 10th

I open my eyes, ears, and heart to listen to my own needs.

October 11th

Each day brings a new chance to thrive.

October 12th

My body has an innate healing power that lies within.

October 13th

I'm not a bad disabled person for grieving the life I

once

October 14th

I do not mourn the life I once thought I'd have.

October 15th

I am creative and strategic when I face new

struggles.

October 16th

Each new day is a fresh start.

October 17th

I find it easy to stay positive.

October 18th

I am open to new treatments but will remember not
to be persuaded by those who want to steal my
money and precious time.

October 19th

I am courageous.

October 20th

Rest is not laziness, Rest is important.

October 21st

Even though I help others I remember to listen to and prioritize my own needs.

October 22nd

Even though there is discomfort inside of me, I love and approve of myself.

October 23rd

I do not let my past define me.

October 24th

I trust myself. I know that all is well.

October 25th

I trust my own intuition.

October 26th

I am in control of the mental atmosphere I create.

Thoughts can be changed and the positive thoughts

I choose are helping me heal.

October 27th

I will let go of stress and tension in my body.

October 28th

I love seeing how healthy habits improve my life.

October 29th

I sometimes give myself permission to mourn the person I used to be.

October 30th

I am the leader of my healthcare team.

October 31st

I do not live in fear.

CHRONIC AFFIRMATIONS

JUDITH S. COPPER

November

JUDITH S. COPPER

November 1st

I have the power to create the reality I want.

November 2nd

My future is bright and full of happiness.

November 3rd

Everywhere I go, I attract positivity into my life.

November 4th

I am grateful for what I can do.

November 5th

It's OK for me to have fun.

November 6th

I give myself room to grow.

November 7th

Pain does not control my life. Only I oversee my life.

November 8th

I am a positive influence on other people.

November 9th

I welcome my pain and invite it in. I am working in partnership with my pain to find peaceful solutions to resolve it.

November 10th

My body is more than capable of supporting me.

November 11th

Thanks for the message brain, but I am OK.

November 12th

I am not alone in my struggles.

November 13th

I choose thoughts that create a healthy atmosphere within and around me.

November 14th

I'm stronger than my insecurities are.

November 15th

If I set my intentions and work towards it, there is nothing that I can't accomplish.

November 16th

My scars prove my strength, not my weakness.

November 17th

My happiness is not tied to my ability to collect material objects or achieve any particular goal, I am a brilliant being just for being here.

November 18th

I will never give up on myself.

November 19th

I take care of myself.

November 20th

My mental well-being is a priority.

November 21st

My body and mind are always striving for perfect
health.

November 22nd

I am patient and kind to myself.

November 23rd

I look for new ways to overcome my challenges.

November 24th

My illness does not limit my happiness.

November 25th

I know my good qualities.

November 26th

I fully accept where I am and am ready to seize this opportunity to grow.

November 27th

Past performance does not equal future success.

November 28th

I trust my ability to make good decisions.

November 29th

I listen to my body and respect the signs it sends me.

November 30th

Happiness is a choice.

JUDITH S. COPPER

December

JUDITH S. COPPER

December 1st

I will make a difference.

December 2nd

All problems have solutions.

December 3rd

I embrace new challenges and try new strategies to work through them.

December 4th

I am capable of so much.

December 5th

My past mistakes have been learning experiences.

December 6th

I breathe light into my pain.

December 7th

I create good health by talking about and thinking about my wellness.

December 8th

I am creating a pain-free future with my thoughts today.

December 9th

My body is more capable than I know.

December 10th

I make responsible choices about my health.

December 11th

My body will bounce back from any affliction.

December 12th

I will improve my health by thinking positively.

December 13th

My efforts help me succeed.

December 14th

My goals are achievable.

December 15th

I will practice self-kindness.

December 16th

I will turn negative thoughts into positive ones.

December 17th

I am not responsible for people's treatment of me.

December 18th

Asking for help is not a weakness.

December 19th

I am still able to practice kindness.

December 20th

I consciously create mental and emotional balance, helping my body's natural healing mechanisms to function.

December 21st

I will prioritize making structures that secure my future and I start today.

December 22nd

I celebrate small wins.

December 23rd

I am the master of my path, the captain of my ship.

December 24th

I find strength in hope and keep a positive outlook.

December 25th

I work out a plan and follow through.

December 26th

I will fight for improvement but will keep a realistic image of my limitations.

December 27th

Investing in my health is one of the best investments I can make.

December 28th

I am so grateful to be alive. I cherish being here.

December 29th

I give myself permission to speak openly about my situation.

December 30th

I do not let myself dwell in my hardships but lead my life in the light of my wins and accomplishments.

December 31st

I know that statistics do not determine my outcome for the future.

JUDITH S. COPPER

Dear reader,

I hope you have gained great strength implementing the daily affirmations in your everyday life and that it has helped you cope and overcome many obstacles and challenges living with your condition.

If you liked this book and found it helpful, then please consider giving it a review on Amazon as it would be of great help with my continuing publishing. It would be much appreciated, and it would encourage me to publish more books on the topic of chronic illness and chronic pain.

Stay strong, I know you can!

Judith S. Copper

JUDITH S. COPPER

Published by

Rittin Books

Made in the USA
Middletown, DE
03 September 2023

37913741R00102